I0428873

the

5

Points

of

POSTURE

Jumper Publications and Media

Disclaimer

The purpose of this book is to empower the reader with knowledge, to educate, informational purposes. This book is not medical advice, but rather the author's personal experience, and is a guide for anyone who wishes to implement said dietary or lifestyle changes at the reader's own discretion. The choice between medical care and self care is completely up to the reader. If you have a medical problem, seek medical care. The author and Jumper Publications and Media shall not be held responsible or liable for any and all damages, loss, or injury, of any kind that may be caused or allegedly caused, directly or indirectly, by the information in this book. Reading beyond this page is the reader's consent to the above disclaimer.

Other Publications

ABC Water and the Number Crunch Diet
a step by step solution to alkaline deficiency and
with a New and Unique approach to weight control

Nontoxic Teeth Whitening and Dental Hygiene System
"Spare me the chemicals, I've switched to FOOD GRADE to
whiten, gargle and brush."

JPM Oral Hygiene Protocol
stop using toxic drugstore mouthwash, discover how to reduce
your gum pocket depth from 3-4-3 to 1-2-1 mm when they probe

12 Changes A Year – Volume 1
the recipe book to the Number Crunch Diet
When you take control of the numbers
you take control of your weight.

NCD Flaxseed Shake Recipe
the Number Crunch Diet method for getting omega 3s
and with three variations so you'll never get bored

12 Changes A Year – Volume 2
the recipe book to the Number Crunch Diet
Begin today and forever be in control of the numbers you're eating.

Vision Is Possible
Improve your vision and get a facelift for free!
an original vision program targeting your Eye Lids

To purchase additional copies, please visit

http://www.CreateSpace.com/4988974

CONTENTS

Edits & Format

You will notice oddities in punctuation, spelling, syntax, and perhaps even semantics, within this book. Feel free to let me know, but some of it is done for brevity or to shift emphasis. I use capitals where I see fit, to grab your attention and make it stand out, and I also remove capitals when I don't think they are deserving of them, or to remove emphasis after first usage, i.e., Pyrex becomes pyrex. And french bread, brussels sprouts, and english cucumbers, are spelled lowercase, as we are not going to "link" a European vacation to our food and eating.

Secondly, I will unhyphenate to create rhythm. Grammatically, two or more words that function as an adjective before a noun are supposed to be hyphenated. That's fine. A million-dollar smile, is the adjective "million-dollar" describing the smile. However, this can get redundant after a while, 1&2 3, 1&2 3, 1&2 3. The noun gets all the attention. But what if you want the adjectives to have the emphasis? After all, the adjectives are the descriptive words. So, I will drop the hyphens to allow the adjectives equal emphasis, and to change the pace of the sentence a bit. So if there are no hyphens, read it slower and evenly, one two three four five six seven. A "step-by-step solution" sounds a bit skippy and simplistic, whereas, a "step by step solution" is said slower and sounds more methodical. Hyphenating two words, or joining two words as a compound word, reduces their individual meanings.

With regard to fastfood, healthfood, and seasalt, it's time for these words to evolve into compound words, so the trend starts here.

There are also some fragmented sentences, subject-verb disagreements, and singular/plural violations. When "correcting" certain of these sentences, they lost their emphasis and punch, so I kept them as is.

In the past I've been guilty of judging other author's sentences, only to reread it with the commas, pauses, and then it made perfect sense. So, if there's a comma, then pause, as you may not get to pause later in the sentence. If there's no comma, then don't pause and read it all as one.

I pose questions, but without question marks. Some are rhetorical, but some are to make you Ponder. Great word. Ponder. If you see a question mark at the end, then it requires an answer. If there's no question mark, then you can just say, yeah, no, or hm.

English continues to change, people using it, customize the language to fit what they want to communicate, emphasize, and to make their point from various angles. It also has to have a variety of melodies and rhythms to keep it from being boring. If you find yourself having to reread a sentence, it may be that it's structured that way for that very reason. So take your time. Don't rush. Let the words digest, so that you absorb the material, and hopefully take some of it and make it a part of your life.

Lastly, you will notice that I customized the headers of every page! This is not something Microsoft Word Starter allows you to do. You can only customize three pages, first, even, and odd. So, to get around this I had to create a Page Break every three pages, and as a result, the last line of some of the pages doesn't "justify" to the edge. So I hope that flipping through the upper corners of the pages will assist you in finding the chapter that you are looking for.

You won't see any citations from scientific studies or PubMed, because at JPM we look to a higher source for our reference.

God Bless!

Enjoy the Journey

Email me if you have a question, or if you just want to comment. Your purchase comes with 1-year free support and photos.

Barry Ogston, B.Sc., CLS, MLS(ASCP)

You have to crunch the numbers to see what you're really eating.

CHAPTER 1

Introduction

Hi! And Welcome!

You are in for a treat! Let me start by saying congratulations up front. Few people take the energy and effort to become polished in every way, shape and form. You've got a wardrobe, you've taken courses, you've examined how you interact with people, and now, you're going to put on the polishing touches. Few people go this route. You are a top performer already. So let's make you even better!

These posture techniques you will not hear anywhere else. Not to be negative about others, but I shake my head whenever I hear or read advice on posture. It is soooooo bad. That "chest out, shoulders back, head up", dear Lord, that is so bad. My techniques are original. I had to create them to get people to learn how to dance. I kept simplifying the dance steps and breaking them down until I scrapped dancing altogether for the first four weeks and said, "I have to fix all your guys' posture before we can begin anything."

The cool thing was, they were okay with it. They knew they couldn't dance, shift their weight, turn, or stand on one leg. They knew they needed the basic basics. Fortunately, these kids and adults had great attitudes, lots of motivation, and plenty of desire, so fixing them was relatively easy. They were good students.

1

1   Introduction

At the end of the season, the adults did a beautiful job performing to "Sail Away" by Enya, the teen class did a great job of "Dancing On The Ceiling" by Lionel Richie, and the pre-teen class proved themselves as dancers when they performed "Da-Doo Ron Ron", but the six-year-old's "Teddy Bear Picnic" number stole the show!

Ah, the 1980s. I do miss those days.

So our five points of posture are:
1. Neck – back of the neck
2. Scapulas – shoulder blades (scapulae, if you prefer that spelling)
3. Ribs – ribcage
4. Pelvis – your hips
5. Big Toe – how you place your weight on your feet

Each of these areas will require a full "class" or chapter, but let me tell you the backstory of an adult student named Judy. She is really an outstanding example of transforming yourself. Not a lazy bone in her body. Do it, discipline, and get it done. Great attitude.

CHAPTER 2

Judy

So I started a community dance program in a small town of 5000 people, mostly farmers. So naturally, walking like a dignitary or a refined person was not what they were all about The women were strong, common sense, good-hearted people. Some of them worked in the city Monday thru Friday, and on weekends they would be involved in renovating a portion of their homes, paint the fence, or drive a truck and haul a boat.

When I first met Judy, she totally did not capture my attention at all. She had a stomach, thighs, big butt, tight jeans, kind of a short torso, and a swayed back. A train wreck, visually. The two that caught my attention as a dance instructor were the tall lean one and the pretty-ish blonde. Boy how I would come to find out that first impressions aren't always right. A lot has to do with the person inside. Their drive and motivation. Judy's body was a diamond in the rough, and over the next 6-12 months she brought it out and transformed herself to the world.

I will never forget how when she took her shoes off and walked across the hardwood floor how much noise she made. Bang Bang Bang Bang as the bottoms of her feet made contact with the floor with each step. I kept thinking, "Doesn't that hurt your heels to walk that hard and heavy." That was just how she walked, loudly, and it never occurred to her. Although I may sound harsh, the truth is, these people were some of the best, nicest, warmest, terrific people I have ever known. I wasn't judging. Be clear about that. I never judged, and still never judge to this day. I was merely noticing things from a dancer teacher's point of view.

The tall lean lady who I thought would be easy to mold was so stiff in her neck and upper back. She had so much muscle tension that I couldn't manipulate her body into the right positions. Every time I tried to fix her head on her neck, it would barely move and she would say it's giving her a headache.

Keep in mind, yes, in the beginning you may experience a headache as you change your posture. Your tense muscles are being stretched and it is going to cause you some pain headaches or other pains in the beginning. This will fade from week to week and will be completely gone, providing you don't go back to your old posture.

So this Judy person worked for a major telephone company, she had a bachelor's degree, and in her mid-40s, she looked pretty much like most women, a big sister, nothing special to look at, but lots of light, brightness, and heart. Now, what if you, I mean you, you reader, what if you could take that nice light, brightness, and cheerful heart and add a fantastic body to it! Think about it. You would essentially be, Celebrity Material.

Very few women, or men, have the whole package. The personality, charm, charisma, and the body, face, and looks to go with it. It's the "whole package" that every man or women is looking to marry. It's Mister Right, or Misses Right. Everything about them is 10-out-of-10 awesome. You want to spend the rest of your life with that person. And lock in with a marriage agreement.

In reality, 80% or more of today's relationships are not like this. In fact, at least half the marriages and relationships out there are two unhappy people staying together just because.

I encourage you, be the first one in the relationship to become "celebrity-like".   Don't wait for your spouse, or don't say to yourself, "Well, he's not so I'm not" or "She's nothing special so I'm not going to be my best either." Forget that. That's lazy talk.

Be a role model and watch the others around you follow along. Or even if they don't, who cares, you just continue to be exemplary, in how you conduct yourself, what you say, and how you look.

Judy did this. Her husband did not. She was a size 13 dress size in the beginning. With dance classes, posture realignment, and her body awareness changing her food choices, she finished the year at a size two. Yes a size two. She said to me, "I've gone from a size thirteen to a size two." And she had. I put my hands around her waist during the class and my thumbs and middle fingers touched. She had a narrow little waist. Remember I said she had a short torso, well, that makes your legs look longer. In the beginning I couldn't see it but now twelve months later, her legs looked long. And because she was a "farm girl" and not afraid of physical work or heavy lifting, she had leg muscles that made her legs look fantastic. Her narrow waist, short torso, long legs, and now her lean body and perfectly-aligned posture, well, she looked like a dancer. In fact, she looked like a ballet dancer.

Who knew that underneath all of those body problems would be the body of a ballerina, I didn't. Now she didn't have the skills and dance ability of a ballerina, that takes years of training, but I could place her leg in an arabesque, hold her upper body up, and put her body in textbook near-perfect ballet positions. As a farm girl, she never had the opportunity to be a ballerina, but at 45 years old, it warmed my heart to see her getting to have a taste of it.

Her primary objective was ladder climbing, she wanted to move up in her job, she wanted to be corporate, executive, and be on the golf course with the male corporate executives. A year later, she was there. She climbed that ladder fast and straight up. Her stories were impressive, although corporate stuff wasn't my thing, I did recognize how high up she was all of a sudden, and her collection of fur coats was growing.

This is an aspect of your career to understand, and that is, as long as you're good, fine, adequate, or very good, you will just stay where you are or move up a notch every five years or so. BUT, once you become polished, the "WHOLE PACKAGE" you get instant recognition, and you are catapulted to the top of your field.

Polished makes all the difference.

You can't just be a seven, eight or a nine, you have to be a ten plus. A celebrity. The Whole Package.

Until you do, you'll just make mild to modest gains in your career. Or you may even go down the ladder as you age and younger people move up. How sad is that. But oh so real.

Judy would take me out for dinner nearly every Friday or Saturday and we ate at fancy hotels and restaurants with beautiful views and then she would always pull out a gift for me before the meal came, and we would finish the evening with an outdoor walk somewhere nice. I considered her my Angel and a true soulmate connection. As time went on though, it became clear that she was too attached, and then I got the call from her husband. I always asked her if John was okay with us having dinner together and she always assured me he was. Well, there came a breaking point. He was jealous and wanted his wife back. Judy was now corporate, stunning, and buying her way through life, and her husband was fat, lazy, and spent all his evenings watching television. How sad. I will say that yes, I do judge lazy people a bit. I just don't have much respect for lazy. He did read books when there was nothing on TV, but the books were fiction, nothing useful, just more mind-numbing escapism.

Here we have two totally opposite people. The wife who is a role model beyond role models, and the husband who is null and void.

You dear reader, be all out, be 100 and 10 percent, be a role model, a celebrity, in your own best way. Never allow lazy and escapism to enter your character. That is my goal for you.

CHAPTER 3

Back of the Neck

So we are going to start at the top and work down, keep in mind that each area will get easier to "feel" and "hold" when all five areas are addressed. That means, the back-of-the-neck position gets easier as the scapulas get fixed, and the scapula placement feels more normal as the ribs get fixed, and the ribs feel easier to hold as the pelvis gets corrected, and the pelvis gets easier to maintain as the weight placement on the feet gets corrected. All that to say, that each of the five will feel more natural as all of the five become properly aligned.

Now just to let you know, that I have been using this posture alignment for more than 30 years and that it applies to both men and women. Although men might think that walking with your chest out and on the outsides of your feet is tough, this posture is very unstable and guys that carry themselves like this are easily pushed off balance and taken down. For you men, I am not saying be like a ballerina, of course not, but bring your strength to the center of your body. This is how punk kids with almost no muscle can be strong, their strength is centered in their body. The more of your energy that is out, away from your body, the more unstable you are. This applies to your emotions and mental energy as well. Bring it all in, to the center, and you will find you'll become an unmoved person, physically, emotionally, and mentally.

Keep in mind, I know nothing about martial arts or meditation or

Buddhism, etc., I am writing this strictly from a dance angle. But centering clearly overlaps with martial arts, meditation, and yoga, although sitting up straight or maintaining a stance are a long way away from *The 5 Points of Posture*, as you are about to discover.

Place your four fingers together, now place them behind your ears and push those two humps on the back of your skull, push them up. Now use the palms of your hands, the thumb area of the palms of your hands, and push those two humps up again, but using the palms of your hands at the padded thumb area. Now, what you should be experiencing is the back of your neck being made LONG. In the front, your chin is likely pushed in and you have a "double-chin" skinfold under your chin.

This is your correct head and neck posture.

Now, I had you overdo the position, overshoot the position, so bring your hands down, shake your head out, move it around a bit, and now find that spot. That spot of the back-of-the-neck LONG.

When I was first taught this by Paula, one of my very excellent ballet instructors, I walked around with a double chin for a few months. Then, one day, it was gone. The back of my neck was long, my head was erect, and there was no double-chin skinfold. Your body will adapt. The double-chin fold will go away. The students I taught also experienced this double chin in the beginning and then in a few months it was gone.

Part 2. Next, place your left hand on the back of your neck. Lift your chin up. Notice how the back of your neck is curved and there is no muscle there, no muscle activated. Now, go to your "Long Neck" position. Over-exaggerate the position. When you over-exaggerate the position, the long back-of-the-neck, you will feel a tendon in the center of your neck that goes straight up into your skull. Tip your chin completely down and you can feel that tendon pop out. Touch it and play with it with your fingers. Press on it and follow it as it goes up the center of the back of your neck up into the center top part of the skull. With your chin down you should be able to feel that tendon sticking up.

The back of your head has three bumps. We already push up on the right and left ones. The third one is the one in the center, up a bit higher on the back of the head, in the center. These three bumps on the back of your head make a triangle or pyramid shape, one on the right, one on the left, one up higher in the center.

They are claimed to be associated with personality traits and I was going to tell you what they were, just for interest's sake, but the internet doesn't say anything about them. Every time I searched, "what are the personality traits of the three bumps on the back of the head", everything comes up cancer and lymphoma, and the couple of phrenology sites don't say anything except that phrenology is bogus science.

Hm. Am I the only person on the planet to search for the personality traits of the three bumps on the back of your head? It seems so, as there is nothing that I could find. And yet it used to be there. Well, one of them was "adhesiveness", how well you stick with something. Anyway, it's not important, I was just going to add it here for interest's sake, but it seems it's all been removed.

Anyway, we are all familiar with those three bumps on the back of our head, that's all I wanted to bring attention to.

That tendon in the center of your neck that pops out when you drop your chin, that tendon goes right up into the center top bump. That's what I want you to feel. Tip your chin down and with your fingers feel that tendon. Follow it from the bottom of your neck vertebrae to the top of the skull, follow it as it goes right inside that center bump. Play around with that for a little while. See if you can get that tendon to pop out. Tense that tendon and make it hard.

It's that tendon that I want you to become aware of. It's that tendon that I want you to start using, start activating. It's that tendon that lifts up the back of your head and LENGTHENS the back of your neck. That tendon right there. That's the key.

CHAPTER 4

That Tendon

99% of the population has no awareness of that tendon. If you start using that tendon you will stand out. Don't worry, the double chin will go away after a while. But if you use that tendon to hold your head, you will instantly stand out from all the rest.

In the beginning I want you to over-exaggerate the position in order to build up the strength of that tendon. Then you will back off a bit and you should be in the correct position. So, go through your day doing an extreme lift of the back of the head and an extreme lengthen of the back-of-the-neck, so that you build some muscle and some awareness back there. Then when you can activate it in the snap of a finger, find it instantly, then you can stop doing the extreme.

I started teaching this group of kids and adults in September, by Christmas they had that muscle built and were using it. However, when I would teach them new steps they would get the feet part, then when I would add the arms, they would lose their long back-of-the-necks. All of their mental concentration was happening at the feet and arm areas and their back-of-the-necks would curl and shorten. All I had to say was "BACK OF THE NECK" and the entire class activated that tendon all at once. It was kind-of cool. I had control over their posture with my words.

I can't be there with you, but as you go about your day, say to yourself, "BACK OF THE NECK" and check yourself to see that that tendon is working and not taking a nap.

Again, 99% of the population has no awareness of that muscle tendon. Get this down solid and you will be a different person.

I wish I could thank Paula more for having fixed my back-of-the-neck and for her taking individual time to physically pull on my head and lengthen my back-of-the-neck so I could feel it. Then she would say, "Okay, right there, that's it, feel that." She permanently changed my life.

When someone positively changes your life for the rest of your life, you look back 30 years later and thank God for those people. The people that bought you a gift or dinner or lunch, well, that was kind and nice of them. But it's the people that positively change your life for the rest of your life. Those people I am most grateful for.

It is my goal that Jumper Publications will positively help people with the types of changes that they take with them and use for the rest of their life. The Oral Hygiene Protocol, the Nontoxic Personal and Household hygiene methods, the diet advice, and the alkalinity aspect. If you haven't purchased any other books from JPM, I recommend any from the list. It's information you won't find anywhere else.

Another thing you can do to feel this long back-of-the-neck position and to feel that tendon working is to lie on your back on the floor, carpet is okay, but a concrete floor is ideal.

When you lie on your back on a concrete floor, the hardness of the concrete seems to push into your body and flatten out your spine and vertebrae. For additional flattening, take a fairly heavy barbell, I use a 50 pound one, and hold it above your chest with straight arms, the beginning position of the bench press. Now, do an abdominal crunch.

The weight of the barbell will work against you and your spine will go click click click and you will feel extremely relaxed and straight and flat.

The posture that we are aiming for will make you less three dimensional and more flat. When you look at most people from the side, they have all these parts sticking out. A lean teenager is flat when you look at them from the side. Think of that cartoon where the cartoon character gets flattened by a road paver. The big round road paver drives over him and flattens him. Or, think of jail bars. Imagine that you have to squeeze through the bars to get out of jail and there is only six inches of space between the bars. Flat. Think flat.

From the front you will look tall and poised, and from the back you will look strong and broad, but from the side you will look not thick. Flat-ish.

This takes us to the next point, point number two, scapulas, the shoulder blades.

Anyways, as you are lying on the concrete floor, pull your chin down, lengthen the back of your neck, almost think of trying to get the back of your neck to press against the floor, then use your hands to feel that extreme position and that tendon should be sticking out and hard/firm. Play around with that position and get to know that muscle, that tendon, and start using it. For most people, that's going to take playing with it and activating it several times a day for several weeks before it becomes natural and automatic, a part of the new you. That's just what you have to do if you want to look tall and pulled-up. You have to activate and build up that tendon strength and mind-muscle connection.

You don't need someone to physically help you find the spot, like I had, and like I did with my students. Just overshoot the position for a while, exaggerate it, to get the feel of the tendon, then when you can activate that tendon and make it work, then back off the exaggeration a bit to the neutral position. Long Back of the Neck.

CHAPTER 5

Scapulas

Now I could say "shoulder blades" but that's two words, and it really doesn't refer to the bones the way scapulas does, and it's the bones that we are going to move.

I would come up behind the students in class and see those shoulder blades sticking out on either side of the spine and I would take my index finger and thumb of my right hand and press a bit on those two bones.

Well, instead of the bones moving, the person would fall forward!

Unbelievable. They couldn't move their shoulder blades. So, I had to modify my correcting slightly. I would put my left arm on the front of their upper chest to block them from falling forward, and then with my right-hand index finger and thumb I would press those scapula bones in and flatten out their back.

Instantly, what happens when you do this is, your arms hang centered on your body. Most people are carrying their arms too far back. It's that "shoulders back" "chin up" advice that everyone's heard so much of.

If you think of a guard or a marine or soldier, there are two postures. One has his chest puffed up and chin lifted up, the other is pulled up at the back of the neck, his chin is level, and his gaze is straight forward. The chest up chin up boot camp soldier is not the correct way to be. But rather, think of the guard, with his chin slightly down, but really it's level, and the back of his neck is tall and long. That's the one you want.

It is interesting how posture that's away from your center makes you unstable and easy to push over. I could push full-grown adults forward with just a mild press of the shoulder blades on their backs.

The other way to get this "flattening" of the back, and the scapulas to move into the back instead of sticking out of the back, is to place your back up against a wall. Bend your knees a bit and flatten out your entire back, lower back, upper back, back of the neck, all against the wall, flat. Allow your arms and shoulders to move forward a bit as you flatten your back and flatten those scapulas.

This should activate your lat muscles, the latissimus dorsi muscles located under the arms. To feel them, give yourself a hug. Place your left hand towards the back underneath your right armpit, and flex the lat and give it a rub, feel it, try to get it to pump up bigger by flexing it harder. Then do the left lat, feeling it with the right hand. For you men, you should be very familiar with this muscle. Women, you may or may not have any feeling there. No worries. You will develop some over time.

Flattening the scapulas causes the arms and shoulders to move forward slightly, in this position it is easy to tighten the chest muscles and expand and flex the lats. Try it. You want this. Absolutely if you are a man, and yes for the women as well.

A female ballet dancer has strong lats, her chest is proud but not lifted, it's flexed, and the back is expanded, via the lats. This will give you women a better figure. Both men and women look better with "hourglass" figures, broad wide shoulders with an expanded back, tapered waist, then muscular legs and butt. It's also a very athletic and "in-shape" look. Again, we are going for "flat" looking from the side, broad tall and proud from the front.

Do this wall exercise several times a day. It only takes 15 seconds to lean your back against a flat wall and find the position and now you know it. Then when you feel yourself losing it, find a wall and get it back. There are walls everywhere so there is no excuse. I can't come up behind you and flatten them so you will have to use the wall. A flat refrigerator door works as well.

While you are against the wall, check the head. Activate that tendon. Drop your chin some and lengthen the back of the neck. Then press those shoulder blades into the back and fan them out to the sides, expanding the muscles under the arms, (the lats), and allowing your arms to come forward and your shoulders to come forward. Your arms aren't really "forward", they are actually centered. Most people, 99% of people, have their arms and shoulders back from the center line of their body. Their lats are completely asleep and inactive, and this puts their lower back in a bit of a sway. And their ribs are sticking out a bit. Some people, men, their ribs are sticking out a lot more than a bit. I'm sure you've seen men like that.

If you look at yourself in the mirror sideways, you will see that your arms are back when your lats are asleep and your scapulas are sticking out. When you place your back against the wall and flatten out your back, flattening those shoulder blades into your back, fanning out your scapulas, fanning out the lat muscles under the arms, you will see that your arms in the mirror are now in the center of your body. Get used to this new posture. It's rock solid, strong, elegant, and confident. Women, don't think that this is too manly a positon, it's not. Most women's upper bodies are so asleep and weak, almost even, pathetic weak, and victim looking. You are not coming across as a bodybuilder, you are coming across as elegant, classy, strong, confident, and dignified. For you men, this is an absolute must. Many of today's young men have upper body posture so relaxed and asleep that they have no "male" presentation or male essence. Man-up and put away the phone. Look and stand and carry yourself like a leader, not a follower.

CHAPTER 6

Home Base

Now, you might be thinking, this posture is too intimidating, I can't walk around with lats activated underneath my arms and my back expanded flat, and my shoulders feeling broad and my upper chest slightly flexed. Well, yes, it is intimidating to some people. Like I said earlier, people will notice you and you will stand out, because 99.9% of the population doesn't have all five of these aspects of posture. Bodybuilders will have the flat scapulas and the activated lats, and they may have a pulled up back-of-the-neck, but they likely have ribs sticking out and their pelvis is likely tipped a bit and their foot placement on their feet is probably out to the sides of their feet. So, if you have all five, you will stand out, and you will intimidate, at first glance.

HOWEVER, you reassure the person or people you meet by being warm fun friendly and nice. Then when you leave, the person says to themselves, "Oh, they're actually a nice person, I judged them wrong." My posture does intimidate, that is true. BUT, I NEVER USE IT TO INTIMIDATE. That's the key. You DO NOT use your strong dignified diplomat posture to intimidate. Be warm and friendly and talk to people, smile and be likeable. The other person will change their prejudgment of you and say "Nice person" "Great Guy" "Great Woman", and they will RESPECT YOU. Strong looking, but personable with no ego.

Look intimidating, okay, but don't **be** intimidating.

You'll be "stamped" with the RESPECT stamp. Or, said another way, they will label you or categorize you as "someone they like, and someone they respect." This person will help you. If it's your waiter, you will get excellent respected service.   If you are checking into a hotel, they will regard you as someone important and call you by your last name or sir, et cetera.

Just don't add a puffed-up attitude to your strong posture. That says EGO, and people don't respect egos. Some people make it their goal to take down people with egos. If you've been with any big-time celebrities, people will say, they are strong, personable, down-to-earth, and nice. They are not puffed up and full of ego and pride. They are stars and it shows, they are attractive, strong, confident, and rich, BUT, they don't come across that way.

That spells respect. You're a star, but you don't act like you're a star.   When you act like you're important or a star or wealthy, people don't respect that, or they do so on the surface only.

So,
1. Present yourself visually as strong, confident, and important.
BUT
2.   Be warm, friendly, likeable, and fun. Or just pleasant and professional if the interaction is brief. And be patient, don't press.

Word of warning for the workplace. As you transform your image, your boss will become intimidated. He or she likely isn't polished. Stand your ground and stick with your new posture. Things may get bumpy as he tries to get rid of you for out-shining him or her. Be pleasant, professional, and without ego, and your boss will blow it. You will have his job. Or you will be snatched up by another department and promoted somewhere else. Like I said, your strong and confident posture will stand out. Top executives will be talking about you in private. Your new promotion is on the table somewhere, just stay cool, maintain competence, be a role model, and set the standard. Let them know it's permanent and real change. After a year or six months, the higher-ups will be convinced you're the real-deal and move you up.

Home Base. Now keep in mind, you don't hold these postures every second of every day. You have your "Home Base" posture and you move in-and-out of it naturally. You don't spend every second in this strong posture. If you are in a meeting or in a job interview then about 80-90% of the time you stay in this posture, showing near total professionalism with a 10-20% human down-to-earth more relaxed posture. If you are having dinner with someone you just met, then 75% of your time you would stay in this posture, and 25% in more relaxed positions. If you are lying on the beach with your spouse, perhaps 40% of your time would be in this strong posture.

The situations will dictate how much you "let your guard down" and be loose and relaxed and how much time you maintain strong confident posture. This posture is your Home Base. You come back to it for centering. You move about and interact, and you keep coming back to the Home Base for centering. When you get home, you can kick off your shoes, lie down on the sofa and turn on the TV and completely chill out. But in public, you maintain your strong confident posture, the amount depends on the environment and the event, always coming back to your Home Base when you leave it for more relaxed, human, connected moments.

This way, your strong confident posture looks very natural. You move in-and-out of it as situations present themselves. If someone brings their kids over to you, you bend down and get human with them, pick them up if that's something you do, then come back to your Home Base. People will see that your strong posture is just natural for you and not something you are "consciously trying" to do. If people sense you are trying to hold your posture, they will see you as a fake and weird. It has to be natural and automatic, and not something you're thinking about.

Other people will notice your strong confident posture, but you yourself don't notice it. You just do it. It's just how you walk, stand, sit, and move. It's just how you are. It's natural and automatic for you.

CHAPTER 7

Ribs

Oh, this is a tough one for people. Why? Because this is where most people breathe from.

Sadly, the wrong place.

Surely you've heard of "belly breathing", breathing from the stomach or abdomen area, your belly. Well, this is better than ribcage breathing or chest breathing, but we are going to go one level lower. Pelvic Breathing.

If you've ever watched a ballet performance, say *The Nutcracker*, you will notice that the lead dancers are doing a lot of physical activity, turns, jumps, more turns, more jumps, and then she finishes with her arm up, a flick of the wrist, and a pop of the head to the second balcony. But it doesn't look like she's huffing and puffing at all. This is the beauty of ballet. She's huffing and puffing alright, but you can't see it because it's happening so low, beneath her tutu. If you were standing next to her you would see her lower ab area, your front bikini area, the area of your "speedo" swimsuit, you would see her breathing from there. At the bottom of the pelvis, just right at the area above the pubic area. That low.

Well, you think it's impossible to breathe that low, from your panty line area, from your bikini briefs area, well, it is possible. And I highly recommend it. If you want to be grounded, this is the way to do it. Place your hands on your hips, low on your hips, and breathe from there, that's deep breathing. That's grounded.

Now, the male ballet dancer does bigger jumps and his entire routine is big jumps and big jumping turns, so you will see him breathing hard, although, if the guy is in good shape, he will finish the routine and he will be huffing and puffing from his pelvis but not in his chest. The audience can't tell. People aren't looking down there to see if the dancer is huffing and puffing. It's their secret. It's how they make it look easy and effortless. Believe me, there is effort happening, dancers just know how to conceal it.

So, think about breathing from down there. We are going to get to that later. For now, it's ribs.

If your ribs are sticking out, you are not flat. So here's what I have people do. Lie down on your back, legs naturally straight. Now exhale and flatten your ribs as you exhale. Contract. Hold it. I know, you can't breathe. If you could breathe from your pelvis then you could breathe in that position. Eventually you'll get it.

You can also bend your knees, feet flat on the floor, and exhale, flatten your ribs, shrink your ribcage. Think, Six-Pack Abs.

As the teacher I would come around to the students and push their ribs down. They had contracted them down, but they were only 50% down. I would push them ALL the way down. FLAT.

This means zero air, completely exhaled. Completely flat ribs. 50% flattened ribs is not enough. You need 100% completely flattened ribs. Exhale everything and flatten 100%, as much as you can, fully flattened ribs, as much as you possibly can. Then hold that position for as long as you can. If it's just a few seconds then it's just a few seconds. Breathe and do it again. Exhale and flatten, then exhale some more and flatten further, and exhale even more and flatten all the way. Hold. Breathe.

Believe me when I say that YOU WILL be able to keep your ribs completely flat and breathe, and even jump, turn, and dance in that position. You just need to transfer your breathing to your pelvis.

When you flatten your ribs and exhale 100% and 100% flatten your ribs, then if you refuse to let your ribs expand, then your body will go down lower to breathe. Essentially, you are forcing your body to breathe lower. Your body wants to breathe, so if you refuse to allow ribcage breathing, by keeping your ribs flat, then your body will naturally go down lower to breathe. So, don't worry. You won't pass out and die. Just flatten your ribs and don't give in. Your body will figure out that it has to breathe lower and it will.

Keep practicing this until it's automatic and natural and that it's your new place of breathing. You will no longer breathe from the ribs.

For the more resistant students I had to go beyond pushing on their ribs. I literally had to straddle their body with my legs, place the palms of my hands on their ribs and push down with all my bodyweight. Picture a paramedic doing CPR, but not from the side of the body, but from the center, having straddled their body. Now, instead of the CPR up-and-down pumping action, I would just push down. If you've spent your entire life with your ribs sticking out and breathing from your diaphragm, just below your pectorals and chest, then changing this is not easy. Many men can't even collapse or flatten their ribs at all, or barely any at all. They've walked around their entire life with their ribs out and flattening their ribs is very unnatural for them, almost impossible. But clearly, the lower you can breathe, and the flatter you can be, the better. The "barrel" stomach and "barrel" ribcage that many men have is not healthy. You may think you're a sexy man, and that the ladies like that big barreled chest and ribcage, but you are going to have to decide what is more important, flat ribs and lower breathing or the macho-man look. That barreled chest and ribs posture is "Heart-Attack" posture. It usually comes with abdominal obesity or overweightness, and poor cardiovascular health. If you watch those endurance runners from Kenya who run 26 miles in two hours, they don't appear to be breathing either.

7   Ribs

They're breathing down low.

So if you can't flatten your ribs on your own with the three exhales, ask someone to push down on your ribs, CPR style, as you exhale, and keep working at it until you can get flat, 100% flat.

CHAPTER 8

Pelvis & Fat Loss

Let's take a minute to review. So far we know there two posture camps, the heads-up chest-out shoulders-back boot-camp group, and the guard group or ballet-dancer group, chin down, (level), back of the neck long, (tendon working), scapulas flattened into the back, causing a concomitant fanning out of the lat muscles underneath the arms, with a second concomitant movement of the shoulders to the center, median line of your body, and your arms not just hanging there but being held at the sides.

And with our ribs flattened with three consecutive progressive exhales, 6-pack abs style, our breathing is forced to drop down to our lower-abs area, our underwear waist-elastic area, our pelvis.

In addition to this strong posture, we interact with people in a friendly warm manner to remove the impression of intimidation.

We also move in-and-out of the posture naturally as we move about and interact with the people and situations in our world, always coming back to Home Base as our center, default posture.

Okay, pelvis. Yes, you know what I am about to say, 99% of the people out there have a slightly swayed or more than slightly swayed pelvis.

Place your right hand behind you and press down at the base of the spine, where your butt cheeks make a "V". Your spine stops at the bottom of that "V" on the exterior of your body. Place your fingers together and place them at the bottom of that "V". Your hand with your fingers together will look like a "V" with your middle finger the longest in the middle and then the pinky and thumb on the outsides. So your "V" shaped hand fits perfectly into the "V" shape of the bottom of the spine butt-cheeks area. Press it down.

When you place your fingers in the "V", you should instantly sense and feel that your pelvis is too high. When you press it down, it becomes vertical, straight, and flat.

Try it.

Now, lock the position with a slight contraction of your butt cheeks. Place your left hand on your lower abs, your bikini area. You will feel your lower abs lift up.

In actuality, what you are doing is:

Using your lower abs in the front to straighten out and push down the pelvis from the back. The front lower abs do the work.

Keep those front lower abs activated and awake, all the time. Whereas you can move in-and-out of your upper body strong posture, you really want to lock in this vertical pelvis and keep it locked, pretty much 80-90% of your day. In other words, you may relax your upper body posture depending on the situation, say, talking to your 90-year-old grandmother, so that you don't come across as strong, but rather soft and compassionate, in this situation with your elderly grandmother, BUT, keep the pelvis straight. There really is no need to relax this area and sway your back, ever. Unless you are going to do a backbend, a back walkover, or a back handspring. Assuming you won't be performing any back-bending gymnastics moves, your lower abs should be always "on", always activated, always pulled up. Keeping your "V" flat and down.

Aside: You have likely notice my writing style for this book. I repeat things and stay them two or three different ways. Some of you may think this is redundant. Not so. As a dance student, my teachers would say something one way to get me to feel the position and the muscles, then they would say it another way, then they would say it still another way. Sometimes it would be the fifth way that they said it that "clicked" for me. Teachers know this. Not everyone grasps something said one way. So as a teacher, you say the same thing in different ways. A great teacher can come up with multiple ways of saying the same thing, and eventually, you get it.

Also, I am violating the rules of grammar again, as I do in my other books, but this one in particular, because it's so instructional. Try to picture us in a studio or class, and I am literally standing beside you and talking and moving and pressing on certain areas. Think of a dance class as you read this. Grammarians need to understand the subject matter that I am trying to get across. And, just like JPM's other publications, there's a certain unique language and vocabulary that goes along with the subject matter.

Once again, you can do the wall flattening of your back, long back-of-the-neck, flat scapulas, flat ribs, and pelvis tucked under a bit and pushed flat against the wall. Bend your knees a little to make it more comfortable. Now I just said "tuck" your pelvis under. You can bend your knees and exaggerate the "tucking" of your pelvis. Then back off and find the vertical spot. Just like we over-exaggerated the pulling down of our chin to feel the position fully. Then back off to neutral and the level chin placement.

You can also lie on the concrete floor, or any floor, and bend your knees, feet flat on the floor, and feel your pelvis and lower back pressed into the concrete floor, flat. This is a very centering, meditative, spiritual, stress-purging position. Fold your arms across your chest, elbows pointing up to the ceiling, in the self-hugging position, and just breathe and close your eyes and flatten out your spine.

Yoga. When I studied yoga, my instructor, Elaine, said that the key to youthfulness is in a flexible spine. The rounding and arching yes, but more importantly, in the twisting of the spine, the spinal twist movements.

I fully agree with that, based on my personal experience. A flexible spine equates to a youthful body. Conversely, an old body is a stiff-spine body.

The exercise for spinal twist is, to sit on the floor, legs out in front of you, now cross your right leg over your left, placing your right foot on the outside of your left leg, right foot flat on the floor. Now, turn your torso to the right, turn your head over your right shoulder, try to look behind you. Hold, breathe, then change sides. Bend your left leg and place the left foot flat on the floor on the outside of your right leg, now turn your torso to the left and look behind you. You can add arm leverage by placing your right arm behind your bent left leg. Some people will then take their left arm and wrap it behind their back. However, when you take your left arm off the floor and place it behind your back, don't allow your torso to shorten and slouch. Stay as tall in the spine as you can. Aim for 100% vertical spine.

You can also bend the straight leg, so if you are turning your torso to the left, your right leg was straight, now bend it under you so that your right foot is on the left side of your hips. It's like sitting down cross-legged, and then raising the left leg and crossing it over the right, then twist and look to the left. It's the Spinal Twist.

For weight loss, the yoga movement is the plough. Sit on the floor with your legs out in front of you, now, roll back onto your back and bring or swing your legs up so that your feet are touching the floor north of your head. You will be balancing on your upper-back and back-of-the-neck and back-of-the-head areas. The backs of your legs will be facing the ceiling, legs together, and your toes will be touching the floor north of your head, depending on what kind of shape you are in. This looks like a plough. You can then relax your knees and bend them and allow your knees to come in towards and next to your ears. Hold and breathe. This works for weight loss because the gut, intestines, and stomach area are forced to compress themselves, shrink. A shrunken stomach means a smaller stomach. This plough movement is the opposite of a backbend. Whereas a backbend or bridge is maximum stretching of the front and maximum arching of the back, the plough is maximum rounding of the front and maximum stretching of the back. Both are great movements to do. But the maximum rounding of the front, via the plough, will shrink your stomach, clear the intestines, and the rest is calorie control, with some exercise, to make the extra skin/fat come off. But this stomach shrinking movement is great for…shrinking the stomach. In fact, step one of fat loss is to eat less so that the stomach shrinks.

Story. One lab where I worked, nine people had had stomach stapling or gastric bypass. Apparently, they have an annual meeting and luncheon. I was told that you can tell who had gastric bypass and who had stomach stapling because the gastric-bypass people would eat too much and have to jump up and run to the bathroom. A paramedic we knew had a gastric bypass three years prior, but he looked 50 pounds overweight.

Moral of the story. No amount of surgery will fix your problem if you don't address the Real Cause.

ABC Water and the Number Crunch Diet

CHAPTER 9

Unmoved

So we have four of the five! Good for you! Don't judge me on the short chapters. This book is not to be read all-at-once. You should be reading three pages, one chapter, then put the book down and practice it. Work on it for a few days to a week. Then move on when you're ready. If you are reading this book straight through, you're missing it. Savour it. Take a little of it and get it into your life. Then when you've got it operational, take another bite of the book and read the next chapter.

Some people are information hogs, eating up information, devouring information, but then they never do anything with it. It's just stored information in their head.

Information is only step one of the process, it's the easiest step actually. Step two is action. Doing it. This is the hard step. You have to find time. You have to play around with it, experiment, practice, and work at it.

This is true for all of JPM publications. They are Selfcare Strategies, or methods, protocols, that you read, and then implement. The ultimate goal or objective it to implement it and make it a part of your life. Dietary and Lifestyle Changes.

Big Toe. This may sound funny, but you really need to relate your big toes. That's more "middle of your body". Medial.

Medial means the same as centering. We are bringing everything about our posture to the center, or the medial, middle plane of the body.

I know a muscular bodybuilder and he is pretty-darn big. Arms, forearms, chest, not so much legs and abs, but big arms, chest, forearms, and shoulders. Well, he walks with his feet turned out to the corners, and on the outsides of his feet. All of his shoes are worn on the outside edges. You know who I am talking about.

Again, a good guy, but his body is unstable. I can knock him and he moves. I just have to give him a good nudge with the side of my body and he steps out. He's completely unstable in his stance. Martial arts people probably look at big-muscled guys like this and think, "I can take this guy down it one move, in two seconds I can have him on the floor."

This brings us to the subject of – Functional Muscle. Bodybuilding is appealing because it creates an appealing attractive body. But all that muscle is not very useful, or functional.   Bodybuilders typically don't perform sports or cycle or run. They might play baseball or football, but not basketball or volleyball. They can't jump off the floor. They are just too heavy with all that muscle. Now visually, yes, done correctly, the body is impressive and "sexy" but functionally, not very useful.

So it becomes a tossup. Do we want a muscled physique that can't jump much or run much, or do we want a functional body?

I say, go for the gymnast body, or the ballet body, or hurdler body, or speed skater. Muscle, but it works for you. It's functional.

So my friend the bodybuilder has unstable posture, even though his muscle and arms are impressive and get him respect. Again, the martial arts guy is looking at my bodybuilder friend as an easy target. Unstable, uncentered, and therefore easy to take down.

I had a pre-employment physical a few years ago, and I put on the gown, and I bent down and touched my toes, and reached back behind me, turn to the right, turn to the left, stand on one leg, stand on the other leg, then, stand and look front. She pushed me. I never moved. She paused and pushed me again but twice as hard, I still didn't move. I could tell she contemplated doing it a third time but then just switched to writing on her clipboard. She was perplexed and irritated that I didn't move. I'll bet I was the first person that she'd ever examined that never moved.

Point being. Strong posture. I am grounded. Solid. No one can move me. Almost like when you see a statue, you go over and try to move it and it doesn't budge. Think about that. The appearance of the statue can be of someone standing and looking forward to the people, and the posture is strong and confident. Leader-like posture. Noble. Not stiff or frozen, but strong and noble.

This brings us to the next two related benefits.

If your posture is strong and unmoved, your emotions will be unmoved. No one can press your buttons. Nice. How would you like to be fully in charge of your emotions? No one can affect you negatively.

Then, with your strong physical posture, and your unmoved emotions, your intellect, thinking, and mindset is unmoved. You are mentally strong and unmoved. No one can press your mental buttons.

Body Mind Emotions

Strong confident unmoved body posture => strong confident unmoved emotional status => strong confident mental status.

The three combined add up to,

strong confident Spiritual status.

You are locked in to a higher source. A God source. A power few people possess.

Why?

Because it all starts with the physical. And most people can't get that area mastered.

If you can't master your physical body, then you can't move on to mastering your emotional and mental states, and then the cherry on the cake, the spiritual.

I've spent a lot of my life trying to figure out the physical body; fitness, diet, muscle building, flexibility, functional muscle, dance skills, and on and on. In doing so, I've come to realize, the reason I placed so much effort into mastering the physical body, is because it's the foundation for mastering the next higher levels, the emotional, mental, and spiritual.

Well you say, that's a bunch of crap, lots of people are spiritual and don't have strong confident posture and fit physical bodies. Yes, to some degree, yes. But, I'm talking 100% solid in your faith and spirituality, 100% unmoved in your faith and belief in a higher power. Some faith or 60 or 70% faith is quite possible, and we see it in preachers and people that we know. But that's not a Master in faith, 100% solidified in their faith, 100% locked into their God source. This is mastery. A whole 'nother level. Many people have some control and unmoved-ness over their emotions, mental states, etc., but to get to 100%, mastery, you have to get the physical fixed. Otherwise, you have a weak link. People, the devil, will see it and exploit it. The devil, in people, will show it to you, and say to you, "Ha!, you're not as unmoved as you thought you were huh!" Mastery is a whole 'nother level. You've arrived. You're 100% locked in and unmoved, physically, emotionally, mentally, and spiritually.

CHAPTER 10

The 10.0

So, male or female, "big toe" really is the correct placement of your bodyweight on top of your feet. It's medial. The center plane of your body.

There's a guy named Christopher Hamel, he jumps off of buildings onto a trampoline and bounces back up and lands on the exact same spot where he jumped off from. It's amazing. It's a 20-foot drop off a building or a parking structure, onto a trampoline at the bottom and seemingly without effort, he flies back up to the top where he jumped from. If you watch how he lands the big jumps, it's "knees together". He's bringing it all in, medially.

When a gymnast does a vault and takes a step back on the landing, she has lost her center, too much force and not enough strength to hold it on the landing, and she takes a step back. A one-point deduction. The perfect 10.0 vault is done with sufficient speed and force, but not so much speed and force that you can't hang on to the landing. The perfect 10.0 vault, the master gymnast, has figured out just the right amount of speed and force, and when she lands, she presses her knees together, almost "pigeon toed" a bit, toes turned in a bit on the landing, knees touching, a low thigh squat, then she straightens up, turns her feet out, brings her heels together, chest up, chin up, arms back, and the crowd jumps to their feet and applauds. She perfectly landed that vault, giving her a 10.0 score. This is a master.

Again, I am not saying you can't be spiritual, or have control of your emotions and mind, but there are degrees to this. The Master is a 10.0, 100%, the gold medalist. The 10.C gets to be on the *David Letterman Show*, the 9.8 does not, the 10.0 gets to be on the front of the *TV Guide*, the 9.5 is not, the 10.0 is recognized as the champion, the 9.9 goes almost unrecognized, or just brief mild recognition. Your pastor may be 95% spiritually refined, but he will always be short of 100% unless he fixes his physical component. If the devil can find an opening in you, he will find it.

There is a very popular preacher on TV and he is excellent, powerful, and Godly. But he's obese. How can you condemn others for sin, when visually, you yourself are clearly in sin, overindulgence of food, gluttony. His credibility would be closer to 100% if he himself was the full package, but until then, he's just a preacher, talking the talk, but not walking 100% of the walk. He has holes.

Many people have experienced that feeling of being "on". At the top of your game. If you are a comedian, then you know when you are "on", if you are a swimmer, your form was perfect and your time was perfect, if you are a father, your household was at peace, everyone was behaving and you were in 100% authority and 100% respected. You are "on".

This happens when the physical is there and "on". Then the emotional falls into place and is in-check. Then the mental is refined, sharp, spot-on, and on track. When this all happens, when these three line up, when the Trinity of Your Being is all "on", the God of all Creation comes rushing in and fills you with the Light of the Universe. You Shine. You Glow. You Radiate. Everything goes right because you are right in all ways. People can see it from across the room. The minute you enter, it's like the Star just entered. What I am saying is, the physical is the foundation for all the rest, your mind, your emotions, and your Spiritual Light.

Your strong confident posture is foundational to that physical foundation. Clearly, you have to be at your ideal weight and have a healthy glow in your face and skin from some cardiovascular exercise, and you have to have some muscle tone so your clothes hang well. In other words, you have to be fit physically, along with the five points of posture.

I had to harp on that a little bit because many people like to dismiss the physical part of their entire package as if it's not a "player" in how they are. Their physical body is their weakest link and so they would rather just try to fool themselves into thinking that, "I make up for it with my strong personality, my calmness, my sternness, my professionalism." Yeah, no. People are looking at your body too. They are just pretending to respect you, when secretly, they don't.

If you are looking to be the master of your profession, your household, your relationship, your life, you are going to have to begin with mastering your physical body.

Sadly, this is extremely rare in our world. And so we have men being tyrants and a..holes to get their way or to get cooperation or respect, and all women know that the best way to manage is to be a bee-och, female dog. The word "lady" isn't even used hardly at all anymore. Nor is "gentleman". But you my friend, are a cut above the rest. Be that star celebrity, and be important and full of authority visually, but show people with your words and actions that you are nice, warm, and a likeable person.

In fact, this is the only way to win when you find yourself up against the a..holes and the bee-oches. Don't try to win on their level. Stay dignified and celebrity-like. People will see the difference. And people love to follow the winners, the celebrity types. The dogs are for the dogs. You're a more elite breed. Never mind them. They will disappear after a while and be out of your hair. Or use the experience to practice and refine yourself. They are testing you. Pass the test. And you win.

CHAPTER 11

Big Toe

So sit in a chair and lift the heel of your right foot off the floor, pressing into the big toe padded area on the bottom of the ball of the foot. Now, lower the heel, but do so through the line of the big toe. Imagine a line going through your foot right through the center of your big toe, down the foot, and up the inside of the leg. This is your center plane of your body. This is your median line.

Now, go back to sitting in the chair with the right heel up and you are pressing into the floor at the padded area of the bottom of the big toe. Now, lift your baby toe off the floor.

Try to lift your baby toe off the floor, and even lift the second toe off the floor.

If your weight is fully being pushed through the center of the big toe, you should be able to lift the baby toe off the floor. Then lift the second toe off the floor, and even the third a little bit.

The point is, get your weight 100% on to your big toe.

Try it with your left foot.

Now stand up and feel your weight going through the two lines. The line going through the center of your right big toe, along the inside of your right foot, and up the inside of your right leg, and the left line going through the center of the left big toe and along the inside of the left foot and up the inside of the left leg.

Get comfortable with this new weight placement.

Once you have it standing, then take a few steps. Walk. Don't turn your toes in or out. Keep the feet parallel. Toes pointing front, straight front. As you walk, feel the pressure, (the weight), go through your big toe, through the big toe lines in the foot, inside of the foot area, and feel the insides of your legs.

This is centered. This is how Christopher the trampoline guy lands his 20-foot trampoline jumps off the side of a building. This is where your strength is.

Imagine "pole dancing". Now take that pole and insert it right through the center of your body. That's where you want to concentrate your muscles. That's your center. Moving away from that center "pole" makes you unstable. You will take a step forward if someone bumps you from behind, or you will take a step back if you're a dancer doing pirouettes.

Walking. Now, fashion models walk a certain way and if you're a woman you may utilize that walk if you want to. It's the walk where you are walking on a line, or try walking on a street curb, or stand on a concrete curb in a parking lot and walk along the curb. This is a great way to check your balance. If you are "off" or stressed out or bothered by something, you won't be able to walk five steps on that concrete curb without falling off. However, if you are calm, and centered, you can walk on that concrete curb perfectly and never need to look down. I do this every so often, to make sure my balance is still on. Then I'll run. Once you've mastered 50-100 steps perfectly, try jogging on the curb, and then running. There's a long concrete-curb area near the beach in Orange County, and I used to go there and literally run on the curb. It's as much mental as physical. You can't be thinking about your problems and walk or run on a curb at the same time. If you have problems on your mind, (stress), you will quickly fall off that curb.

Try it. It's good for your balance, and it's an easy way to check to see if you are centered – physically, emotionally, and mentally.

Now for you men. This is not the way you will walk. Not if you want to have friends. So you can still walk with your weight going through the center of your big toe and along the line in your feet and up the inside of your leg, just separate the distance between your feet. In other words, walk with your feet "hip width apart". For me, it's about four-and-half inches apart. When I look down at my legs, or if I look at my legs in the mirror, they are coming straight down from my hips. So for you men, feet parallel, placed 4-5 inches apart, or 6 inches if you are six-feet tall, HIP WIDTH apart, whatever that distance is for you, then place the weight of your steps through the center of the big toe, and follow that line along the inside of the foot, and up the inside of the leg.

Women, this would look funny for you. So place your feet one or two inches apart and walk that way. Or if it's 5pm on a Friday you can walk one foot in front of the other on a line and tell the world, "Look at me! I'm a hottie!" You get the idea.

The point is, male or female, the weight placement is the same for both. Then masculinize your walk by walking with your feet hip-width apart, or feminize your walk by walking with your feet one-inch apart, or do the fashion-model walk if you so choose and walk on a line. Feet are parallel for all walks, male, female, fashion model. Men, you may think that walking with your toes turned out is manly, but it's not, it's more monkey if anything. If you want to use it at 5pm on Friday to pick up babes at the bar, well, make it a style walk, and not your everyday walk.

Tip. If you run or jog and your knees hurt the next day, then run with your feet hip-width apart. It's harder to do, as landing your feet directly underneath you is easier, but that directly-underneath-you position is angled, and that's what's hurting your knees. Run hip-width apart. Start with 2-3 inches apart, and work your way up to 4-5 inches apart. Your legs will become more powerful this way also. Hurdlers run this way, feet hip-width apart.

CHAPTER 12

Summary

So there you have it. The only five things you need, to change the entire way people view you.   Long back-of-the-neck, use that tendon, activate it, chin level not raised, scapulas, shoulder blades, flattened into your back, not poking out of your back, thus making your lat muscles flex and come alive, and they fan out to the sides underneath the backs of your arms, and at the same time your shoulders move forward a bit to be more medial, through the center of your body, and your arms are carried and held in a natural position by the activation of your scapulas, lats, and front pectoral chest muscles. Your ribs are flat, exhale and flatten them, three times, to get 100% flat ribs, this forces your body to go lower for air, down to the pelvis, the hips, and then you flatten the "V" at the bottom of your spine, top of your butt cheeks, and flatten that, but really it's activating your front lower abs, pulling up the front of your lower abs to vertical-ize the pelvis. Then you draw in your mind an image of a line going through the center of your big toes and along the insides of your feet and up the insides of your legs, and that is where your weight placement should be going, feet parallel, and 1-2-3 inches apart if you're a woman, and 4-5-6 inches apart if you're a man.

You move in-and-out of your posture naturally so as not to make it look forced or held, and you come back to home base as your default. Being friendly and likeable so as not to give people the impression that you are an egomaniac or a psychopath or a fake.

This will work, I've been using it for more than 30 years. The only downside is that the people above you won't know how to get the edge over you. But that's okay, you'll be above them before too long. Or they will rise up, realizing that they have to "up" their game. That's really the ideal goal. It's not a competition. You set the bar, and never lower it, they either rise up, or they play like an animal and dig their own grave. Either way, it doesn't impact you. You are Unmoved.

Then, as you continue to polish and refine your physical appearance, along with courses in your profession, practicing your professionalism and craft every day, one day you may just find, you've got it all mastered, you're a 10.0, the light of the universe coming down and through you, flooding every cell of your body, it's evident, you're "on" and people can see it. Everybody wants you. You're a star. A celebrity.

Judy went from the middle of the ladder to the top of the ladder in her career in about 18 months. Visually, she went from a 5.0 to a 10.0. She looked like a million bucks. Her dresses hung straight down, her narrow waist, from the bottom of her spine-hips to the top of her spine-head she was straight and tall, an expensive blouse, jewelry, high heels to go with her legs and leg muscles, long legs with her short torso, the hair, the smile, everything, she was a star in her world. Not on television, but in your own world, aim to become a star, not for the glamour or attention, but for just being and living the best life you can be. That's what I found most amazing. She went from average to incredible. Unlike her husband, Judy was an inspiration for everyone around her, a complete life transformation. She attributed her success to me fixing her posture, but I told her, "You did it. I just did my job."

Chapter Endnote
With regard to John, of course everyone has some redeeming quality, and the spotlight is not for everyone. John was very supportive of his wife, and it may well have been that he was the "wind beneath her wings".

PREVIEW
from the
ABC Water and the Number Crunch Diet

As you know, the recipes for the NCD are being published under the titles, *12 Changes a Year* – the companion guide to the Number Crunch Diet. It may take up to a year to get them written as it will comprise about three volumes. In the meantime, you can get your pH paper testing set up and determine your current alkaline stores. The recipes read like a book and include additional information that I've discovered about diet, lifestyle, health and selfcare. I look forward to seeing you over there!

To join my mission in providing people with safe, effective, affordable, selfcare protocols, send someone you know to www.abcwaterandthenumbercrunchdiet.com. Tell them to take the Quiz!! Thanks for your support! God Bless.

Jumper Publications & Media
From Advice to Results

I almost forgot! (again, not really) to tell you!

If you liked this shake recipe be sure to check out

TCY
12 Changes a Year
Vol 2

for the NCD ORANGE SHAKE!
It makes 9, and I often repeat the recipe midweek.
And whey protein – but not from powder.

BUY THE BOOK!!
IT'S GOOD STUFF!

FREE REPORT #1

JPM Mouth Rinse Protocol™

In the highly competitive world of publishing and creating a following, a reader base, you've always got to give your audience something for free. This way, if the book was not quite what they thought it was worth, the "free" item will hopefully make up for it. Keep in mind, I price things according to what I would pay for them and according to other things. People pay $250 to see a sporting event, but squawk about the price of information that can positively affect their health for decades to come. A one-night stay in your average hotel room while on vacation can cost $179, and it's long gone. Someone told me he sold a used fishing lure on eBay for $400. What's really going to help you on your journey?

As a lifetime seeker of self-improvement, I have never thought twice about the price if I knew it would benefit me. I left Timothy Ferris, author of *The Four Hour Body*, a 5-star review, even though I had to read all 572 pages of his book to get two things out of it. But, it's two things that I didn't have before I read the book. A person with a lot of these Gold Nuggets is miles ahead in the game of life than someone who just goes along never seeking information. So, there's your good advice. And if you are curious to know what those two things are that I got from his book, stay tuned!

Okay, I'll tell you.

This may not be new to some of you but it was to me.
1. Glut Ham Raises – totally works the backs of your legs.

Not just the hamstrings but the calves and butt as well. Attempt to do 12-15 slow reps in 60 seconds and you will feel it the next day. Best bang for your Back-Of-The-Leg buck. However, for erectors, inner hip muscles, I still like single leg "rocking" deadlifts.

2. MED – Minimal Effective Dose
It's best explained like this. Water comes to a boil when it reaches 100 degrees celsius. Adding more heat, more energy, doesn't make it boil more. Applying this to exercise, it's the old "Stimulate Don't Annihilate" rule. Do one set to failure and that's it. Stop. You're done. Let your muscles break down and regrow bigger. It works. And the best part is, you keep cortisol levels under control. Heavy workouts can zap your body for days, especially when you're over 50!

So this is why *ABC Water and the Number Crunch Diet* is priced like a BMW. It's Revelation Information. A synergy of dozens of books and specialties, to create a completely new book. Selfcare.

So your free report is about "How To Improve Your Gums And Teeth". Two words. Hydrogen Peroxide.

But not so fast. There's the detail.

JPM Mouth Rinse Protocol™

I have to give credit to my brother for this one. He is 62, has never had a cavity, and 33-years ago his dentist told him that he doesn't need to keep coming to the dentist, that, "You're your own dentist."

Now, how many people do you know of that have been told by their dentist that their personal dental hygiene is so good that they are their own dentist and that the dentist actually tells them to stop coming to the dentist? I only know of one. My brother. And he has fantastic teeth and gums, and he's 62, retirement age. What was his secret weapon all these years. Hydrogen Peroxide.

I recall a coworker telling me she had so many dental problems and she was so upset about them. I told her to rinse with hydrogen peroxide. She came back the next week with a big smile on her face, all that anxiety that she had was gone, and she sincerely thanked me profusely. She was smiling bigger and I could tell her gums were looking better already.

Lack of Attached Gingiva. Nobody wants to hear their dentist or dental hygienist say this. Gingiva just means gums. Lack of attached gums, means you have pockets. You know, like when they do the probing of your gums, 334 333 233 432. They go around your teeth checking the pockets of your gums at three locations on each tooth, cheek side and tongue side. Bleeding and pockets means GINGIVITIS. Gum Disease. Bad News.

But there's hope. You can, in my experience, and obviously in my brother's experience, have healthy gums by rinsing with hydrogen peroxide. But there's some do's and don'ts, so keep reading.

I will give you the whole protocol that I do so that you can set it up for yourself at home and begin today to drop those pocket measurements from four and three millimeters to two and one millimeters, and yes, it is possible to have zero mm pockets. Zero mm pockets means you have 100% fully-attached gums to your teeth. My brother has this. You can tell when he smiles. He's got solid gums that are gripped solidly on to his teeth. No pockets. No recession. No Lack of Attached Gingiva.

Of course we have all asked him where he got the idea to rinse with hydrogen peroxide. His answer is brilliant.

"I just thought, well, I'll rinse with hydrogen peroxide."

You see, you don't have to be a doctor to know things, or a PhD, or a licensed blah blah blah. My brother is none of those things. Yet he's a genius when it comes to oral hygiene. AND, the most notable part of his discovery is, It Just Came To Him. Like a thought. Or a revelation. He already had a million-dollar smile, so he was thinking about how he could maintain it and improve on it so that he could have that million dollar big teeth square jaw smile for his whole life.

Imagine having perfect teeth and gums and you haven't been to the dentist in 33 years. In the ABC NCD book I talk about not paying too much attention to crossover double-blind placebo-controlled scientific studies. For some things, the obvious answer is right in front of your face. Just look and believe it. I don't need a study to prove to me that hydrogen-peroxide rinsing can transform bad gum tissue into healthy gum tissue and reduce pocket depth. I use it and it does it. Every one of our family members uses it. We are all following my brother's oral hygiene protocol.

So, here's what you do.

Initial Setup. Buy 8 bottles of 15oz Lea & Perrins Worcestershire sauce at the supermarket. Transfer the liquid to a one-gallon container, or discard it, then proceed to thoroughly rinse the bottles and scrub off the labels. Now you have eight 15oz glass amber bottles with tight-fitting screw caps. The amber color will prevent light from degrading the H_2O_2 into water, and the screw cap will prevent oxygen from getting inside and reacting with the H_2O_2 and converting it into water. So your hydrogen peroxide will stay potent. Also, if you haven't already read my website, we here at JPM and ABC NCD are Plastiphobes. We avoid plastics for eating and for anything that will go in our mouth or used on our body. The HUGE one is, never microwave food in a plastic container, and the lesser evils are, storing the shampoo you use on your head in a plastic container. Replace the plastic containers in your kitchen and bathroom with glass wherever possible.

So, this 15oz bottle is ideal and you'll see why as we go along.

Next. Buy a gallon of hydrogen peroxide. I get mine at Smart & Final supermarket and restaurant-supply store, $8. It's the most economical, $1 per 16oz. And a gallon will keep you from running out. Fill your eight worcester bottles full to the top, to the brim, and then cap them. The bottle holds 16oz exactly, so you have the exact amount needed to fill all 8 bottles to the top. If the bottles were really only 15oz, then 8x15=120oz, and a gallon is 128oz, so you would have 8oz left over. BUT, lucky for you, I have already figured out the perfect bottle.

The other reason for using this bottle is because it has a small mouth. You want to be able to control the amount of hydrogen peroxide entering your mouth as you take a "swig". A wide-mouth bottle will have you pouring in too much H_2O_2 into your mouth. This is important because:

1. Hydrogen peroxide is for external use only. Don't Drink it.
2. If you get too much in your mouth, and it makes contact with the back of your throat, your throat will dry out and you'll end up with a raspy voice.

That brings us to the Technique.
Pucker your lips and use your tongue to control the liquid as it enters your mouth. When you have about a tablespoon of hydrogen peroxide in your mouth, half an ounce, close your lips and use your cheeks to swirl the liquid around your teeth and gums.

DON'T LET IT TOUCH THE BACK OF YOUR MOUTH

You will have a raspy voice and dry throat if you do.

H_2O_2 IS NOT FOR GARGLING

I will tell you what to use for oral gargling at the end. Your Second Free Report!

So with the H_2O_2 in your mouth, swirl for 30 seconds minimum or 60 seconds maximum. Any less than 30s and you're not doing it long enough for cleaning action to occur, and any longer than 60s and it's no longer doing anything because it's all deactivated, reacted.

Until you get comfortable with this technique, keep your chin down. The natural reaction is to gargle as you are swirling. Don't.

KEEP YOUR CHIN DOWN in the beginning. After a month, the habit should be solidified and you will be able to keep your head in its natural upright position and multitask or stare at yourself in the mirror as you swirl. Are you looking HYA??

Place one of your worcester 16oz hydrogen-peroxide bottles in the shower for your morning oral-hygiene routine, and place the other in the medicine cabinet above your bathroom sink for your before-bed oral-hygiene routine.

16oz will last about one month, 1T, or half an ounce, times 30 days. So, once a month you will start a new bottle in the shower and a new bottle in the medicine cabinet. This is why eight bottles and the one gallon of hydrogen peroxide is the way to do it. When you run out, you just grab another bottle. Two bottles a month means that your eight bottles will last you four months. So every 4 months, or 16 weeks, 3 times a year, you have to pick up a gallon of H_2O_2 and aliquot it into your eight bottles. This is your system.

I gave a bottle to a friend and he freaked out because his gums were foaming up. I said, "Yeah, your gums are foaming up because your gum lines are dirty." He did it twice a day and on the third day they just foamed up a small normal amount. He thanked me profusely.

And I do mean profusely. People are amazed at how amazing this works for reversing bad gums and for making them look that healthy pink color. And no more sensitive areas after a while.

And I've NEVER heard this anywhere. I honestly believe that when this goes viral, mainstream, because of its effectiveness, that the originator was my brother, back in the 1970s, when something, God maybe, inner Divine Intelligence maybe, said, "I think I'll try rinsing with hydrogen peroxide."

You heard it here first. But the credit goes to my brother Ken!

FREE REPORT #2

JPM Mouth Wash Protocol™

This next one, I will take credit for. And that's the mouth rinse for gargling, aka, mouth wash.

You know, I've never liked using mouthwash. Whenever I tried it, you know, the typical brand they advertise on TV that starts with the letter L, my eyes would get red and my mouth would burn and I'd spit it out and ask myself.

"Why does mouthwash have to feel so toxic?"

Well, fast-forward to the modern world and we now know that IT IS TOXIC. It's loaded with toxic cancer causing birth defect inducing hormone disrupting CHEMICALS!

You will never convince me that thymol, eucalyptol, methyl salicylate, menthol, alcohol, benzoic acid, poloxamer 407, and caramel, are safe and essential for oral hygiene. Salicylate is aspirin. Why does mouthwash need aspirin? To calm the inflammatory effect from all the chemicals.

And that "alcohol", well, it doesn't say if it's ethanol, the drinkable one, but it could be isopropyl alcohol, rubbing alcohol, the poisonous one, or it could be a mixture of the two. Dr. Hulda Clark in her book, *The Cure For All Diseases*, states that she detects isopropyl alcohol contamination everywhere in our lives because the food industry uses it to sanitize. So the next morning they start up the food-processing machines and all that isopropyl alcohol residue ends up in the food. In trace amounts and randomly, yes, but when you are getting exposed to it from every angle, it begins to build up in the body. She stated in her book that every single cancer patient is toxic with isopropyl alcohol.

There's a group of people who bash her books, and I am not saying she was 100% spot-on with every word she wrote, no person is, and she often said when interviewed that, "We haven't discovered that part yet." But her 604-page book is packed with information and it's the reason that today you hear about pollutants, contamination, chemicals, toxins, detox, and purity. I highlighted and underlined more than half of the book and it took me six months to read it.

So although I take credit for this mouthwash, I really need to give credit to the late Dr. Hulda Clark and *The Cure For All Diseases*. You see, vodka is food-grade alcohol. It's the only food-grade alcohol. And alcohol is a good germ-killer, sanitizer, cleaner, and antiseptic.

JPM Mouth Wash Protocol™

Buy a 1.75 liter bottle of vodka, 40% alcohol by volume, not 25%.

I used to buy the Heritage brand 1.75L 40% vodka at Albertson's supermarket for $9.99, $8.99 on sale, plus tax, but the bottle is plastic.

Plastiphobe

So now I buy the "UV" brand 40% vodka in the 1.75L glass bottle. It's $16.99 at Albertson's, but other grocery stores stock it as well.

I spent a while deciding which glass bottle of vodka to go with, and the UV brand won, as the glass is clear, the shape is smooth, and it has indentations at the back for your hand to grip it. Nice.

40% is too strong for gargling so you will want to dilute it 50/50 half-and-half with water. Go to the healthfood store and buy a few bottles of bottled water in glass. Drink the water and remove the labels. I use Voss brand 400mL cylindrical glass water bottles with screw caps. Nice and classy looking when you get the label cleaned off. Place the bottle on your scale and turn it on. Add 200 grams of vodka, then add 200 grams of water. Voila, 20% vodka.

This is your mouthwash for gargling.

As with the worcester bottles, buy eight Voss water bottles so that you have some ready-to-use when you run out. I use this 20% alcohol to rinse my mouth after meals during the day, along with flossing and brushing. For toothpaste I use Trader Joe's/Tom's brand, with Fennel, Propolis and Myrrh, lavender color on the box.

Tom's brand has been around for a long time and back in the 1980s is was the only Health Food toothpaste. In the 1990s they used to put the PURPOSE for their ingredients on the toothpaste box. So, they had a list of about six ingredients in one column, and the purpose for each ingredient right across from it in another column. They stopped doing this. Now they just list the ingredients, and shockingly, GLUTAMATE is ingredient number seven. This is why I don't use toothpaste that frequently. Glutamate, Excitotoxin, is in my Health Food toothpaste. Terrible.

JPM Oral Hygiene AM Protocol™
Brush – toothpaste
Floss
Mouth Rinse – 1T H_2O_2 30-60sec
Mouth Wash – 20% vodka gargle & rinse 10-15sec

Throughout the day and after eating:
Brush – no toothpaste
Floss
Mouth Wash – 20% alcohol gargle and rinse

JPM Oral Hygiene BB Protocol™
Before Bed same as AM

Hard/Firm toothbrush if my tongue feels a gritty film anywhere. Scaling tool once a week on anterior lowers (minerals in my saliva tend to precipitate on the backs of my lower teeth). And I use one of those long Oral B-60 toothbrushes to clean my tongue AM and PM. A lot of people neglect their tongue hygiene.

If you don't already own one, a Must-Have is an electric toothbrush. Hand brushing simply can't compare to the fast vibrating movement of an electric toothbrush. Philips Sonicare $35, works great. I keep one in my car. (No that's not weird.)

I am not as fortunate as my brother in that I still go to get my teeth cleaned every 6-12 months, but my hygienist and dentist always remark at how good my gums look, and how clean my teeth are. Apparently, a lot of teenagers have poor gum health and oral hygiene. Soft drinks! It's liquid sugar. The NCD considers soda pops as poisons, especially acidic colas. They're Anti-Nutrition. Health destroying.

Recall from the ABC NCD that – No amount of good can counter the bad you expose yourself to daily. You've got to eliminate the bad. In the old days, I can remember coke being used to remove the corroded-metal buildup from the posts of a car battery. And it worked good. Think about what it's doing to your teeth and gums.

As a final note, my next project is to discontinue using 3% topical hydrogen peroxide from the body-care aisle, and order 35% food-grade hydrogen peroxide from www.purehealthdiscounts.net. Then, just dilute it to about 3% by adding 1.5 ounces of the 35% H_2O_2 to the worcester bottle and then filling it to the top with water. See *Nontoxic Teeth Whitening and Dental Hygiene System*

And as another word of caution regarding the use of hydrogen peroxide as a mouth rinse.

IT'S NOT RECOMMENDED IF YOU HAVE METAL FILLINGS.

The H_2O_2 will, on a small scale, dissolve the metal, and those metal atoms can then be absorbed into your bloodstream via the capillary beds underneath your tongue, causing you to auto-intoxicate yourself over time.   But if you have metal fillings in your mouth, your saliva is doing the same thing to a lesser degree 24-hours-a-day 7-days-a-week.   If it was me, I would still do the hydrogen-peroxide mouth rinse AM and PM, as the benefits of having attached gingiva and healthy gums outweighs the risk of trace amounts of metal dissolving, getting into the bloodstream, and traveling to various locations within the body.   Best advice is to have them removed and redone with composite, PLASTIC!

As a benefit to using the H_2O_2 mouth rinse AM and PM, you'll have nice white teeth!   Peroxide is the active ingredient in most teeth whiteners.

Hope You Enjoyed This.

Jumper Publications & Media
Your First Choice for Selfcare

Once you've set up these two oral hygiene protocols and begin to see the benefits for yourself, why not hit the website and purchase a copy for a friend or family member, boss, coworker or your employees. For $30 you could purchase 10 copies and hand them out as "thank-you" tokens to people you know. Remember, it's fully copyrighted ISBN 978-1502489142 so making copies and free distribution is illegal – and bad Karma!

Leave a Review

Without giving away the contents, "spoilers", recommend this publication and leave a review so that someone else might benefit from it too. Thank you.

www.amazon.com   Search: 5 points of posture

Subscribe to my YouTube Channel
www.youtube.com   Search: Number Crunch Diet

Be sure to send me an email so I can periodically keep in touch with updates and new Selfcare Strategies – and discount offers on new items (yes, more than books!) (a simple and effective weight-loss device) (a weightlifting "device" that I use EVERY time I work out) and don't forget the recipes! – TCY.

abcwaterandthenumbercrunchdiet@mail.com
Privacy – your email address will not be used for anything other than by Jumper Publications and Media.

FOLLOW-UP

You know, I've never liked the idea of brushing with baking soda because I've had in my mind all these years a picture of my dad brushing his teeth with the white-and-blue box of Arm & Hammer baking soda, and I assumed it was the one from the cleaning products aisle, which has contaminants and is too abrasive.

So, that glutamate in my toothpaste, and the fact that something in me, my Divine Intelligence, is telling me it's not good, has led me to rethink the baking soda for brushing.

Well, here's what you do. Buy baking soda in the BAKING aisle at a good-quality supermarket, I buy mine at Trader Joe's Market and it's USP, United States Pharmacopeia grade, the highest grade you can buy. To a 16oz glass jar, add the entire contents of the baking soda, use it to brush your teeth. Just wet the bristles and touch the powder, brush for two minutes, works great. Just the right amount of abrasion, not too rough not too mild. The food-grade USP baking soda in the baking aisle is so finely ground it's like a light soft powder, Perfect. The baking soda also gives your body a slight amount of bicarbonate, sodium bicarbonate, for alkalinity. See *ABC Water and the Number Crunch Diet* for the significance of alkalinity to good health, energy, and being ailment free.

So the JPM Oral Hygiene Protocol™ becomes,

1. food-grade or USP-grade baking soda to brush
2. 3% topical or food-grade hydrogen peroxide for gum lines
3. 20% food-grade vodka to gargle

The hydrogen peroxide and the baking soda will whiten.

If you do buy the 35% hydrogen peroxide, dilute it to 6% instead of 3% for a super-powerful teeth whitener! However, if you just be consistent and do the hydrogen-peroxide mouth rinse protocol AM and PM every day, you won't need more whitener. The 3% twice a day works perfectly. Happy Hygiene!

Saliva vs Urine pH

Top Ten Reasons Why Saliva pH Is Worthless When Compared To Urine pH For Acid-Base Analysis

#10 Small Volume – small tiny volume samples don't represent the whole

#9 Difficult to Obtain – the procedure is to bring up saliva and swallow, 2x, then use the third one for the test, too hard to obtain

#8 Poor Reproducibility – when you retest your saliva sample, you will likely get a slightly different color (reading)

#7 Poor Accuracy – if you collect a second sample, it will likely give you a different reading than the first

#6 Bacterial Contamination – bacteria from your mouth will interfere with the test

#5 Food Contamination – food from your mouth will interfere with the test

#4 Spoon Contamination – the surface of the spoon that you collect it on is going to affect your small sample

#3 Viscosity – saliva is too thick and results in faded or dual colors of the test pad (or paper)

#2 Difficulty Reading – the color doesn't "lock in" so you can take a reading, it tends to change shades through a range

#1 Your Salivary Glands have ZERO to do with Acid-Base regulation. Try Kidneys.

Your kidneys are running your body's alkaline status.

And your alkaline status is the secret they don't want you to know.

JPM Oral Hygiene Protocol

This publication is the introduction to JPM. If you paid $2.99 for the kindle version or $4.99 for the paperback version, then you basically paid for the two protocols, the 20% vodka mouthwash, and the Secret Weapon, H_2O_2 gum-line cleaner. You will notice advertising for the other publications. Don't be upset. You got your $3-5 worth. The same cost as for a venti mocha latte, that's long since gone. The information in this publication will be with you for you to use for the rest of your life, every day.

So, why not take the ABC NCD Quiz!

The first half of the book is all about alkalinity. The secret aspect to your health no one, but a few, will talk about. However, no one covers the subject better and more comprehensively than in ABC Water™. The second half is the Number Crunch Diet™. No recipes, but lots of good sound information on diet. You will learn a lot, as no one discusses it the way I do. I brag a bit about the book, because it's really a great book. It's a compilation of nearly 100 books that I've read. But more of a Synergy, a new approach.

The recipes can be found in *12 Changes A Year* and you can see a sample on www.abcwaterandthenumbercrunchdiet.com

The title *Nontoxic Teeth Whitening and Dental Hygiene System* begins with the two chapters you just read, but includes a one-of-a-kind food-grade teeth whitening system, if you feel you need more whitening. It also includes a commentary on fluoride. Wouldn't you like to know if fluoride's something you should be doing, or something you shouldn't be doing?

So put your thinking cap on and let's start the Quiz!

It's good for you!

Pick the correct answers – There may be more than one

1. A urine pH of 5 is telling you
   a. about your blood pressure
   b. that you're tired
   c. about your alkaline reserves
   d. to see a doctor
   e. that you're healthy and fine

2. Urine pH testing is routinely performed by licensed
   a. social workers
   b. clinical laboratory scientists
   c. respiratory therapists
   d. fitness advisors
   e. nurses and doctors

3. The cost of one month of urine pH testing is _____ the cost of open heart surgery (CABG).
   a. 1/10
   b. 1/100
   c. 1/1000
   d. 1/10,000
   e. 1/100,000

4. The opposite of metabolic acid is dietary
   a. phosphates – found in meats and cola drinks
   b. bicarbonate – found in packaged foods
   c. caffeine – found in green tea
   d. bicarbonate – found in fruits and vegetables
   e. bicarbonate – found in oils and fats

5. Information can be of which types
   a. true
   b. incomplete

c. false

d. clouded

e. secret

6. "Natural Flavor" on a food label is
   a. natural flavor extracts from plants and fruit
   b. glutamates, MSG, altered salts
   c. chemicals that make you addicted to the product
   d. generally safe and good for me
   e. not something I need to worry about

7. During World War II, the people who failed to act early
   a. suffered
   b. died
   c. lost everything
   d. became victims
   e. made it through unscathed

8. Compensating means
   a. saving for retirement
   b. eating foods that lift your mood
   c. doing something to mask something
   d. brushing it out of your thoughts
   e. pleasing others and being a do-gooder
   f. all of the above

9. The reason(s) people are fat
   a. they're born that way
   b. they don't make their own meals
   c. hereditary – handed down from your parents
   d. my body just won't lose fat
   e. they don't see the numbers in what they're eating

10. The "Cheat Day" is
    a. a great way to get food cravings satisfied
    b. required to reset my fat-burning hormones
    c. a 2-8 step backwards day
    d. works well for most people long term
    e. is a popular "trick" that you should buy into

ANSWERS

1. A urine pH of 5 is telling you
    a. about your blood pressure – No, but there is a relationship (see Chapter 24)
    b. that you're tired – No, but there is a relationship (see Chapter 20)
    c. about your alkaline reserves – YES! Get to know your alkaline status by reading this book.
    d. to see a doctor – No, but it can lead to that.
    e. that you're healthy and fine – One number tells you little, 35 numbers a week tells you a lot. Get to know your urine pH.

2. Urine pH testing is routinely performed by licensed
    a. social workers – no
    b. clinical laboratory scientists – Yes, 99% of all urine testing is done by a CLS.
    c. respiratory therapists – no
    d. fitness advisors – no
    e. nurses and doctors – Doctors do perform urine tests in their offices, but they are not looking at urine pH with much depth.

3. The cost of one month of urine pH testing is _____ the cost of open heart surgery (CABG)(a bypass, "cabbage").
    a. 1/10 – no
    b. 1/100 – no
    c. 1/1000 – no
    d. 1/10,000 – Yes. You can test all of your urinations for about

$1 a month (see Chapter 11). A cabbage would run you at least $10,000.

    e. 1/100,000 – no. But I believe the potential to save yourself $100,000 in medical treatments is very possible.

4. The opposite of metabolic acid is dietary
   a. phosphates – no, phosphates contribute to acidity
   b. bicarbonate – no, bicarbonate yes, but not from packaged foods
   c. caffeine – no, caffeine is a drug, most drugs are acidic
   d. bicarbonate found in fruits and vegetables – Yes!
   e. bicarbonate found in oils and fats – no, oils and fats are not sources of bicarbonate

5. Information can be of which types
   a. true – Yes, this is a bit what your life is all about. Finding the truth about things.
   b. incomplete – aka, partial truths or half truths, aka, "spin". Do you find your head spinning when you go for fancy medical treatments?
   c. false – lies, yes lies. Don't call them untruths. Lies are Lies. When people lie it's your job to call them on it. Otherwise, "ya got no backbone".
   d. clouded – blurry, muddied, confusion. I could write "scientifically" but I would just make you confused and half lost. How does that help you.
   e. secret – Now we're talking. When they say "buy this stock" you've got to be a moron to buy it. The payoffs and the winners are kept secret, shared through word of mouth.

6. "Natural Flavor" on a food label is
   a. natural flavor extracts from plants and fruit – Well, they would like you to think that, but that's far from reality.
   b. glutamates, MSG, altered salts – Yes, often this is the case.
   c. chemicals that make you addicted to the product – Yes

Absolutely
d. generally safe and good for me – don't buy that line
e. not something I need to worry about – you make your own choices in life

7. During World War II, the people that failed to act early
Referring to this is grim and bleak. But there are people suffering and dying every day because they failed to act early. You could say that WWII is still happening all around us in the United States of America today. My book can help you not to fall victim to this death and suffering. So that you make it through your life, unscathed.

8. Compensating means
   a. saving for retirement – no, but I have seen people who are just a little too attached to their portfolios, compensating?
   b. eating foods that lift your mood – no, but food is commonly used to compensate
   c. doing something to mask something – Ah-Ha, Yes.
   d. brushing it out of your thoughts – no. It's okay and healthy to let go of thoughts, just be sure you're not avoiding your issues.
   e. people pleasing – reward seekers may be compensating
   f. all of the above – no, just C. Go back and read C again.

9. The reason(s) people are fat
   a. they're born that way – don't give me that
   b. they don't make their own meals – Bingo! This is key.
   c. heredity – your fat jeans are because of your fat genes – no I don't think so
   d. my body just won't lose fat – I hear you. There is not a lot of good help out there. Luckily, you've found the right place.
   e. they don't see the numbers in what they're eating – Yes. And person D above just needs to look at food mathematically (and read the book).

10. The "Cheat Day" is
   a. a great way to get food cravings satisfied – Wrong. I'm a testimony of getting rid of food cravings. See Chapter 38, 39, 40, 41.
   b. required to reset my fat-burning hormones – Wrong. If you get your macros right, your hormones will cooperate just fine.
   c. a 2-8 step backwards day – On page 84 of *The Four Hour Body* the person states that he gains 4.4 lbs on his cheat day. Then he loses it. Can you say "moody"?
   d. works well for most people long term – After reading dozens of diet books, I could not find one that worked long term, so I made my own. It's called the Number Crunch Diet.
   e. a popular "trick" that you should buy into – The Number Crunch Diet isn't about cheating. Although it's full of useful "tricks" that I came up with and use daily.

You'll be miles ahead of the average person after a while.